Allergic

Natural remedies for seasonal allergies

DR. MARTIN DOSIHMA

Copyright © 2022 CP Print All rights reserved

The characters and events portrayed in this book are fictitious. Any similarity to real persons, living or dead, is coincidental and not intended by the author.

No part of this book may be reproduced, or stored in a retrieval system, or transmitted in any form or by any means, electronic, mechanical, photocopying, recording, or otherwise, without express written permission of the publisher.

ISBN: 9798320452883
Imprint: Independently published

Cover design by: Art Painter
Library of Congress Control Number: 2018675309
Printed in the United States of America

DEDICATION

This book is dedicated to all battering with one form of seasonal allergies or the other; this eBook will help bring lasting solution to your fear and problems. Its another new beginning towards getting lid of all seasonal allergies

INTRODUCTION

For seasonal allergy relief, there are a number of treatments to help you feel better, from prescription and over-the-counter medications to natural remedies.

In this book we will cover, all natural remedies to help you live an allergy free life.

Are you tired of the annual battle with sneezing, itchy eyes, and that perpetual stuffy nose that just won't quit? Well, you're not alone! Seasonal allergies can turn the most beautiful time of the year into a full-blown tissue-fest, leaving us feeling like we're auditioning for a role in a never-ending allergy commercial.

But fear not! This book is here to be your trusty sidekick in the fight against those pesky pollen invaders. Welcome to "Natural Remedies for Seasonal Allergies" - your ultimate guide to reclaiming your spring and summer from the grips of hay fever!

Inside these digital pages, we're diving headfirst into the all natural remedies that can help you find some much-needed relief. From time-tested herbal remedies to lifestyle tweaks that you can use and can make all the difference, we've got you covered.

So, if you're ready to bid farewell to the days of being at the mercy of pollen counts and now hello to a clearer, happier season, then let's embark on this uncovering together, we are here to guide you. Say goodbye to those itchy eyes and let's get ready to enjoy the outdoors fresh air without fear!

Let's jump in and start feeling better, naturally we got you covered.

Stay tune as we unfold all the treatments and precautions to take to feel better and better you must be my friend.

CHAPTER ONE

What causes seasonal allergies?

Many people are allergic to pollen. Their reactions are strongest during spring, summer and fall, when the amount of pollen in the air is high. Mold is also a common seasonal allergen.

What are the symptoms of seasonal allergies?

- Congestion, including nasal congestion and cough
- Itchy eyes, ears, nose and throat
- swollen eyelids
- skin irritation
- Low energy level

Relieve seasonal allergies with these tried-and-true techniques.

Spring means flower buds and blooming trees — and if you're one of the millions of people who have seasonal allergies, it also means sneezing, congestion, a runny nose and other bothersome symptoms. Seasonal allergies — also called hay fever and allergic rhinitis — can make you miserable. But before you settle for plastic flowers and artificial turf, try these simple strategies to keep seasonal allergies under control.

Reduce your exposure to allergy triggers

To reduce your exposure to the things that trigger your allergy signs and symptoms (allergens):

- Stay indoors on dry, windy days. The best time to go outside is after a good rain, which helps clear pollen from the air.
- Avoid lawn mowing, weed pulling and other gardening chores that stir up allergens.

- Remove clothes you've worn outside and shower to rinse pollen from your skin and hair.
- Don't hang laundry outside — pollen can stick to sheets and towels.
- Wear a face mask if you do outside chores.

Take extra steps when pollen counts are high

Seasonal allergy signs and symptoms can flare up when there's a lot of pollen in the air. These steps can help you reduce your exposure:

- Check your local TV or radio station, your local newspaper, or the internet for pollen forecasts and current pollen levels.
- If high pollen counts are forecasted, start taking allergy medications before your symptoms start.
- Close doors and windows at night if possible or any other time when pollen counts are high.
- Avoid outdoor activity in the early morning when pollen counts are highest.

Keep indoor air clean

There's no miracle product that can eliminate all allergens from the air in your home, but these suggestions may help:

- Use air conditioning in your house and car.

- If you have forced air heating or air conditioning in your house, use high-efficiency filters and follow regular maintenance schedules.
- Keep indoor air dry with a dehumidifier.
- Use a portable high-efficiency particulate air (HEPA) filter in your bedroom.
- Clean floors often with a vacuum cleaner that has a HEPA filter.

CHAPTER TWO

Try an over-the-counter remedy

Several types of nonprescription medications can help ease allergy symptoms. They include:

- **Oral antihistamines.** Antihistamines can help relieve sneezing, itching, a stuffy or runny nose, and watery eyes. Examples of oral antihistamines include cetirizine (Zyrtec Allergy), fexofenadine (Allegra Allergy) and loratadine (Claritin, Alavert).
- **Corticosteroid nasal sprays.** These medications improve nasal symptoms. Examples include fluticasone propionate (Flonase Allergy Relief), budesonide (Rhinocort Allergy) and triamcinolone (Nasacort Allergy

24 Hour). Talk to your health care provider about long-term use of corticosteroid nasal sprays.

- **Cromolyn sodium nasal spray.** This nasal spray can ease allergy symptoms by blocking the release of immune system agents that cause symptoms. It works best if treatment is started before exposure to allergens. It's considered a very safe treatment, but it usually needs to be used 4 to 6 times daily.
- **Oral decongestants.** Oral decongestants such as pseudoephedrine (Sudafed) can provide temporary relief from nasal stuffiness. Some allergy medications combine an antihistamine with a decongestant. Examples include cetirizine-pseudoephedrine (Zyrtec-D 12 Hour), fexofenadine-pseudoephedrine (Allegra-D 12 Hour Allergy and Congestion) and loratadine-pseudoephedrine (Claritin-D). Talk to your health care provider about whether the use of a decongestant is good for treating your allergy symptoms.

Rinse your sinuses

Rinsing your nasal passages with saline solution (nasal irrigation) is a quick, inexpensive and effective way to relieve nasal congestion. Rinsing directly flushes out mucus and allergens from your nose.

Saline solutions can be purchased ready-made or as kits to add to water. If you use a kit or home-made saline solution, use bottled water to reduce the risk of infection.

Homemade solutions should have 1 quart (1 liter) of water, 1.5 teaspoons (7.5 milliliters) of canning salt and 1 teaspoon (5 milliliters) of baking soda.

Rinse the irrigation device after each use with clean water and leave open to air-dry.

Alternative treatments

A number of natural remedies have been used to treat hay fever symptoms. Treatments that may improve symptoms include extracts of the shrub butterbur, spirulina (a type of dried algae) and other herbal remedies. Based on the limited number of well-designed clinical trials, there is not enough evidence to demonstrate the safety and effectiveness of these remedies.

Results of studies of acupuncture have shown possible limited benefit, but the results of studies have been mixed.

Talk to your doctor before trying alternative treatments.

When home remedies aren't enough

For many people, avoiding allergens and taking nonprescription medications is enough to ease symptoms. But if your seasonal allergies are still bothersome, don't give up. A number of other treatments are available.

If you have bad seasonal allergies, your health care provider may recommend that you have skin tests or blood tests to find out exactly what allergens trigger your symptoms. Testing can help determine what steps you need to take to avoid your specific triggers and identify which treatments are likely to work best for you.

For some people, allergy shots (allergen immunotherapy) can be a good option. Also known as desensitization, this treatment involves regular injections containing tiny amounts of the substances that cause your allergies. Over time, these injections reduce the immune system reaction that causes symptoms. For some allergies, treatment can be given as tablets under the tongue.

CHAPTER THREE

What natural remedies are there for seasonal allergies?

First, gargling with salt water can soothe a sore throat.

It may also be helpful to clear your nose and throat of potential allergens, such as mold or pollen. To do this, use a saline nasal rinse or a Neti bowl.

If you are using a flushing device, such as a Neti pot, you must use and clean it properly.

When should I see a doctor about my allergies?

Talk to your health care provider about the best way to manage your seasonal allergies, especially if you are considering using an over-the-counter medication or dietary supplement. Keep in mind that some over-the-counter medications and supplements may interact with medications or other supplements, or have their own side effects.

Any serious respiratory problems should be treated by a medical professional. However, if you are trying to treat your symptoms before seeing a doctor, do not use more than one type of over-the-counter medication at a time. If you have an existing condition, such as coronary heart disease, high blood pressure or diabetes, or if you are pregnant or breast-feeding, consult your doctor.

Distinguishing between allergies and a cold is key to relieving your symptoms. Most natural remedies for seasonal allergies are available immediately, but if your symptoms worsen, see your doctor.

Home remedies to relieve allergy symptoms

How to forget about red eyes, mucus and respiratory problems caused by grasses, pollen or dust without medication

llergies are reactions driven by the immune system **to** exposure to a specific component, which may be a **food**, a chemical substance, or environmental factors. The reaction and degree of severity are determined by the type suffered. Although they usually do not have many additional complications, some can be fatal and **extreme caution** should be taken.

Allergic diseases in Spain **affect 30% of the population**, around 16 million people. Among those allergic, approximately half are allergic to plant pollens. The ones that cause the most allergic problems in descending order are: **grasses, olive, cypress, salsola, plantain and parietaria** .

As spring has approached, the sale of antihistamines has grown considerably. Although last year was a very tough season and affected even people who had never suffered it before, forecasts indicate that **this year it will be less intense** . "Those allergic to grass **pollen** will face a mild spring in the Canary Islands, the Mediterranean coast and the northern area, moderate in the center and Andalusia and intense in Extremadura," reveals Dr. **Ángel Moral**, president of the Aerobiology Committee of the Spanish Society of Allergology and Clinical Immunology (SEAIC).

CHAPTER FOUR

Pollen level in the air: check the allergy intensity in your province

The Spanish Society of Allergology and Clinical Immunology has presented a new website where the level of allergens present in the atmosphere is reported.
Runny nose, sneezing, red eyes, itchy throat. The arrival of spring brings with it the inevitable appearance of **pollen allergies** . To check the state of the air in terms of the level of allergens present in the atmosphere - grasses, olea, cupressaceae, plantago, amarantaceae, platanus, urticaceae and betula - the Spanish Society of Allergology and Clinical Immunology (SEAIC) has presented its new page. "Being able to know the levels of atmospheric pollens, their seasonality, the concentration peaks and the duration of the pollen season is very useful in environmental health to try to reduce the effects of pollen allergies. The tools that provide this data are the pollen collectors of the SEAIC Aerobiology

Committee," explains Dr. Ángel Moral, president of said committee.

The Aerobiology Committee is one of the many scientific committees of the SEAIC. Its main objective is to promote research in the area of aerobiology - that is, the study of pollens and fungi found in the air - and pollinosis - **allergic diseases caused by pollens**. It has a network of collectors that is made up of **54 aerobiological stations** to obtain detailed information on pollen levels in all those areas where they are found. The members of each of them have been duly trained in the capture and recognition of the most important pollen types from an allergological point of view.

This committee has been counting pollens since 1973, although it was in 1978 when it began to be done uninterruptedly throughout the year. The counts are provided through the website **completely free of charge and without restrictions** for all those interested, whether professionals or patients, as long as their use is not for commercial purposes. The new website is the update of the one launched in 1999, a virtual initiative that to date has been consulted by more than 1.3 million people.

Polenes.com uses a **color code** similar to that of the traffic light: it categorizes the alert level — **low-green, medium-orange and high-red** — in the different provinces by type of pollen. The new system also allows comparisons to be made between dates and by pollen varieties. "Sometimes, **patients with allergies** access generic information that is very lax and imprecise, so they end up treating their disease with symptomatic medication instead of preventive medication and do not go to the specialist," warns Dr. Joaquin Sastre, president of the SEAIC.

Also in mobile application

The PolenControl application, endorsed by the SEAIC, has also been recently updated. It now offers the possibility for the allergist and/or pharmacist to receive information **via email about the symptoms presented and the medications used during the pollination season without having to go to the doctor's office or pharmacy.** The data to show the levels of the most allergenic pollens are extracted from the website www.polenes.com

Without a doubt, it is a useful tool that provides comfort to the patient. In any case, as Dr. Joaquín Sastre concludes, "although new information and communication technologies have come to facilitate the control and monitoring of the disease of allergic patients, they **should never replace the role of the allergist** ."

CHAPTER FIVE

The foods that cause the most allergies

The foods that cause the most allergies are milk, eggs, shellfish, nuts, wheat, legumes, soy, fruits and fish

If it is not a seasonal allergy but is pathological, it may make many aspects of your daily life difficult and at the same time carry a high socioeconomic cost. As stated by Dr. **Joaquín Sastre** , president of the SEAIC, immunotherapy or allergy **vaccination** should always be considered a first-rate therapeutic tool in the management of allergic patients. "It provides a significant reduction in the total health costs induced by allergic **respiratory** disease , reducing all expenses," he explains.

But for people who unnecessarily suffer from these seasonal or specific reactions, there
are easy, **natural** and **home remedies** that will help relieve the symptoms:

Spring allergies

Quercetin is a natural bioflavonoid that helps stabilize mast cells and **prevents histamine** release . It is also a powerful antioxidant that can reduce inflammation. It is best to use it as a long-term remedy and take it about 4-6 weeks before allergy season. So you should add foods such as onion, oats, apples, grapes, broccoli, tea, spinach or garlic to your **diet.**

Nettle leaf is another natural antihistamine that can be very effective because it blocks the body from producing histamine. It grows in many places and can be made into tea (be careful when picking it). They can be combined with other types of leaves (mint or raspberry) to make it more refreshing.

As for **honey** , there is still much to study about its effects on allergies, but there is a theory that if you ingest several daily doses (three tablespoons, possibly a month before the allergy season) of this product (which be local), it is a **natural**

vaccine for your pollen allergy. As it is produced in the area where you live, your body gets used to and adapts to the allergens in your environment. Eat it alone or with other foods but do not cook or bake it because it will lose the pollen it has due to the high temperatures and then it will be useless.

When we have redness, one of the most common mistakes is to rub our eyes to relieve them. But be careful because it could hurt you more.

Drinking **juices** rich in ascorbic acid or vitamin C will help to have a stronger immune system to combat the attack of these external agents.

To eliminate mucus

Apple cider vinegar is a very old remedy and is recommended for a wide variety of health conditions. For allergy symptoms and heartburn it is very successful. The theory is that its ability to reduce mucus production and cleanse the lymphatic system makes it very useful. To avoid attacks, drink a glass of water three times a day with a tablespoon of this unfiltered organic vinegar.

Salt water is great for clearing nasal blockages caused by mucus. It is true that there are some inhalers that work wonderfully and unclog instantly, but since it is not advisable to abuse them, you can prepare a homemade solution on your own. You will only need a cup of warm mineral water and a tablespoon of salt. **Mix these ingredients well**, making sure the **water** is not too hot, and pour a teaspoon into each of your nostrils, breathing in this liquid. Due to the antiseptic properties of salt and the effect of warm water, you will be able to effectively reduce nasal congestion and drain mucus. If you gargle with this water (30 seconds, 4 times a day), you will also eliminate them from your **throat**.

Infusions **of mint, fennel, lemon balm or eucalyptus** (although if you can boil them and inhale the vapors, even better) help improve breathing. Breathe in the steam for at least 10 minutes twice a day and you will see how you can eliminate mucus faster than you think. Additionally, taking a **hot shower** will cause the water vapor to loosen **nasal blockages** and drain them.

Eye redness

It is a very delicate organ and some allergies can lead to conjunctivitis and this can be the trigger for something more serious. When we have **irritation or redness** , one of the most common mistakes is to rub the **eyes** to feel a sense of relief. However, doing this will not relieve the inflammation, but could cause more damage.

To avoid more problems, you can use **chamomile** , because the components of this herb are ideal for giving our eyes their normal tone. You will need to leave the bag with this plant in a container with hot water, then put it in the refrigerator and let it rest for 24 hours. Then we can use it 3 times a day, soaking a cotton ball with this **infusion** or putting the same bag directly. Apply directly to each eyelid and leave it on for a few minutes.

Rose water **, carrot, cucumber, or potato** are other remedies to prevent redness. You can cut some slices of these foods (that are cold) and put them in each eye, this way you will cool them down, once they become warm, replace them with others. As for the petals of this flower, they have a calming and cooling action ideal for **redness** . Dip a cotton ball in water and place it on each eye for ten minutes.

Food Allergy

They are an exaggerated response of the immune system due to the consumption of a particular food. As **Montserrat Fernández** , from the Allergy Service of the San Carlos Clinical Hospital in Madrid, points out, the normal response of the immune system to foods is to tolerate them. However, in some cases it generates an altered response that can cause, when people consume certain foods, harmful effects and reactions by the immune system that give rise to food allergies. The foods that most frequently cause allergies are milk, eggs, shellfish, nuts, wheat, legumes, soy , fruits and fish.

Rashes, itchy skin, nasal congestion, sneezing, watery eyes, vomiting, nausea or diarrhea are some of the most common symptoms. **There is no prevention as such for a reaction due to an allergy to a** specific food. If it happens to you, you should go quickly to the emergency room to have the reaction subsided. **Drinking** plenty of water is very important and if you mix it with two tablespoons of **oatmeal**, it is very possible that you will slow down the process.

CHAPTER SIX

This is why you may develop an allergy this spring

30% of Spaniards suffer from them, but in the last decade the number of allergy sufferers has grown and is expected to continue doing so in subsequent years.

n Spain, some eight million people are allergic to pollen, a number that, according to allergology specialist at the University of Navarra Clinic, **Carmen D'Amelio**, has gradually increased in the last decade. And although specialists point out that the intensity of these **allergic reactions** to plant pollen will be moderate, there are those who believe, like Dr. **Bill Freeland**, an expert at the London Allergic Clinic, that it will affect even those who have never suffered this type of alteration, and They will increase in virulence and duration in the most susceptible people.

But why are sneezing, itchy and runny noses more frequent than they should be? According to Dr. D'Amelio, a person's **genetic predisposition** has a lot to do with it, but there are also other reasons, including increased pollution.

Something that Dr. **Victoria Cardona**, head of the Allergology service at the Hospital de Valle de Hebron in Barcelona, agrees with, pointing out the ways in which pollution can enhance allergies: "On the one hand, the polluted air we breathe **irritates the mucous membranes** of the pharynx, nose and lungs and makes us more susceptible to suffering from them; on the other hand, diesel particles function as pollen carriers and, in addition, a synergy is created between them and the pollen that maximizes their allergenic effect.

The climate is also another important factor and, above all, the climate change that has caused, according to Cardona, that the pollination season of plants such as the shade plantain, very common in cities like Barcelona or Madrid, is extended beyond the four weeks, so allergies also last longer. On the other hand, the **conditions of a territory** affect allergies; Thus, while in northern Europe it is common to develop an allergy to grasses, in the south there is a great variety of native species and a greater number of allergic reactions.

As many pollens as people

There are around 30 different types of pollens that cause allergies and it is possible that we may be allergic to more than one type.

Thus, grass and olive pollen are more common in certain regions, such as Andalusia, and register their most intense levels in May. "For example, allergy to cypress pollen lasts from January to March and that of **plantain** , with a high incidence in Madrid, starting in March," concludes D'Amelio. However, the symptoms are not the same for everyone and will depend on many factors, such as the patient's susceptibility or if they develop rhinitis, riconoconjunctivitis or asthma. Bronchial.

BEST SEASON

www.ingramcontent.com/pod-product-compliance
Lightning Source LLC
Chambersburg PA
CBHW051536240526
45471CB00020B/3078